D1398502

# Fad Diets

by
## Linda Kita-Bradley

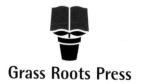

Grass Roots Press

*Fad Diets* is published by
Grass Roots Press, a division of Literacy Services of Canada Ltd.

Phone:       1-888-303-3213
Website:     www.grassrootsbooks.net


ACKNOWLEDGMENTS

We acknowledge the financial support of the Government of Canada through the Book Publishing Industry Development Program (BPIDP) for our publishing activities.

We acknowledge the support of
the Alberta Foundation for the Arts
for our publishing programs.

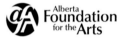

Copy editor:      Judith Tomlinson
Photography:      Susan Rogers
Book design:      Lara Minja, Lime Design Inc.

**Library and Archives Canada Cataloguing in Publication**

Kita-Bradley, Linda, 1958-
        Fad diets / by Linda Kita-Bradley.

ISBN 978-1-894593-80-9

        1. Readers for new literates.  2. Readers—Reducing diets.
3. Readers—Nutrition.  I. Title.

PE1126.N43K58254 2008        428.6'2        C2008-901990-3

Printed in Canada

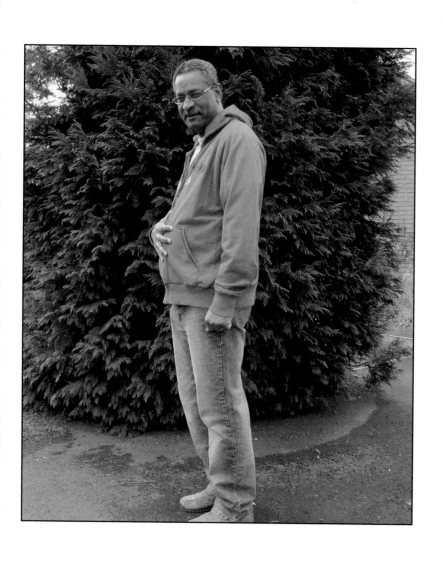

This is Al.

He wants to lose weight.

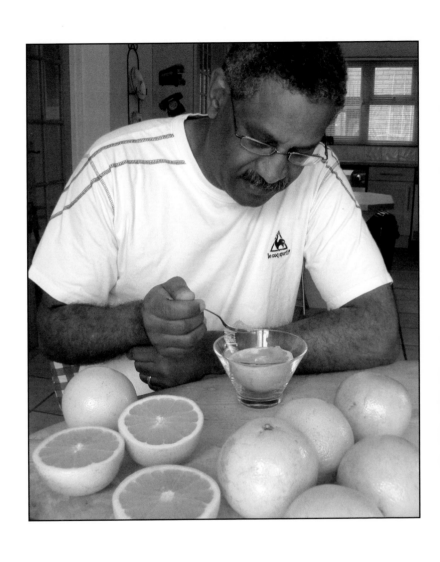

Al tries a grapefruit diet.

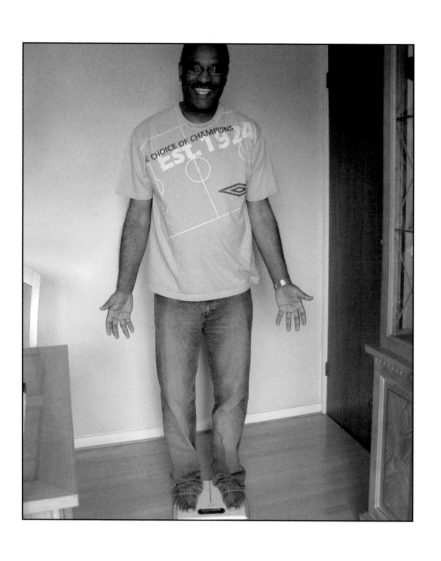

Al loses five pounds in three days.

He is happy.

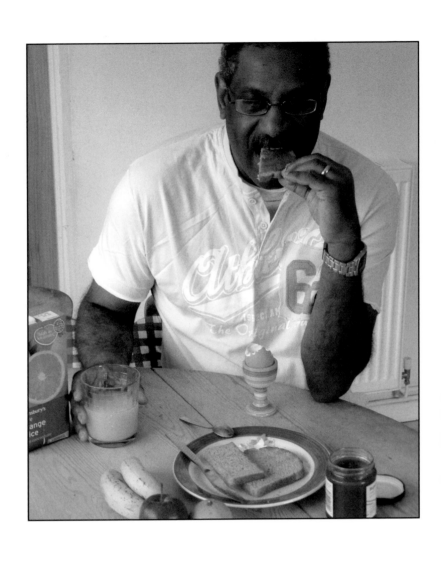

Al starts to eat other food.

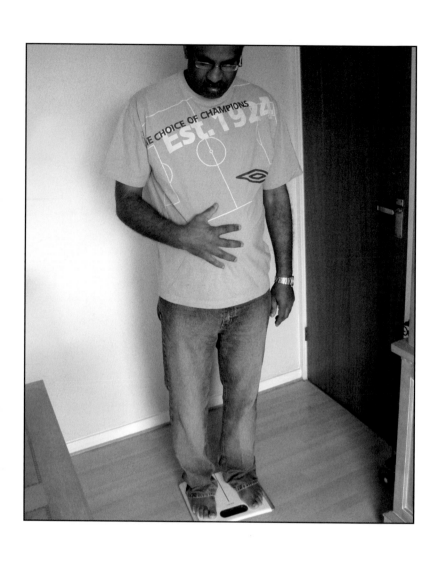

The pounds come back fast!

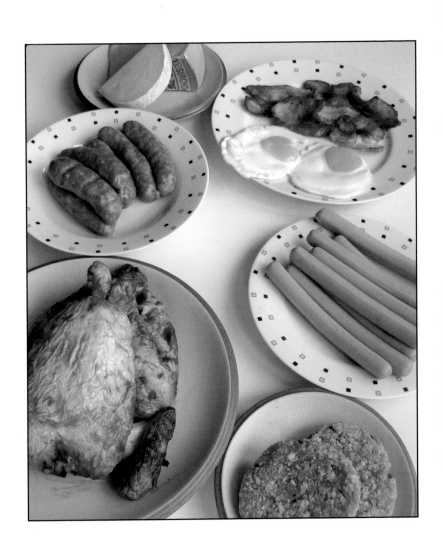

Al tries another diet.

He eats only meat and fatty food.

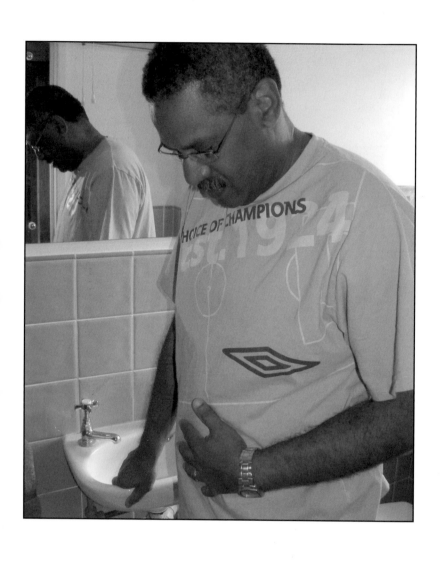

Soon Al has stomach problems.

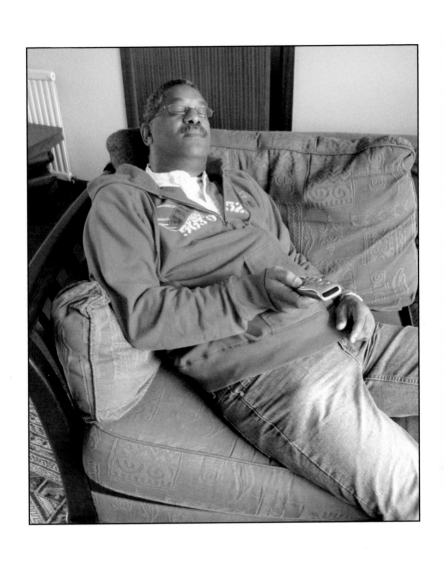

Al feels tired all the time.

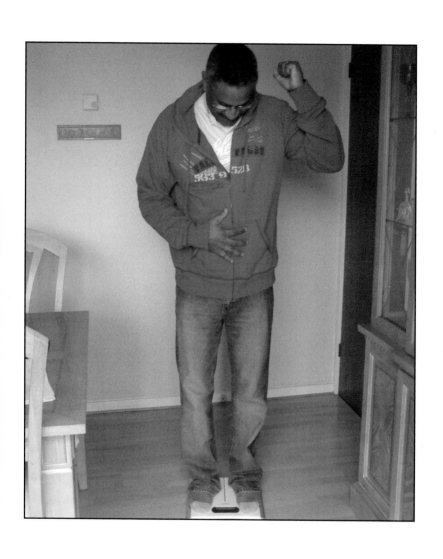

But he loses ten pounds
in two weeks.

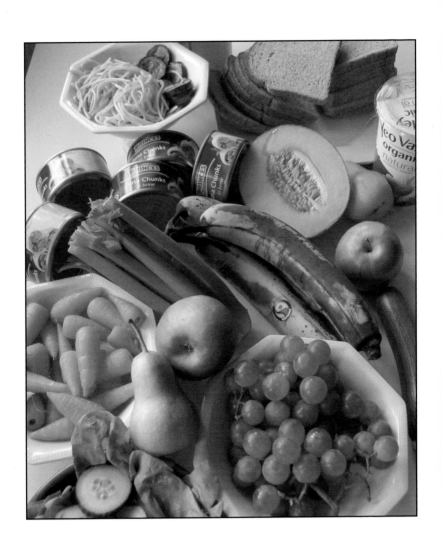

Al starts to eat other food.

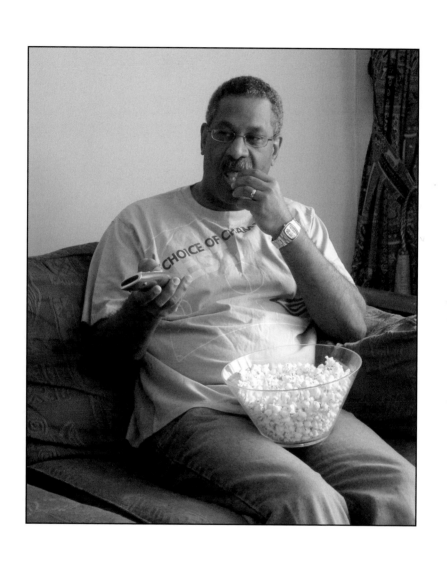

He feels much better.
He is not so tired.

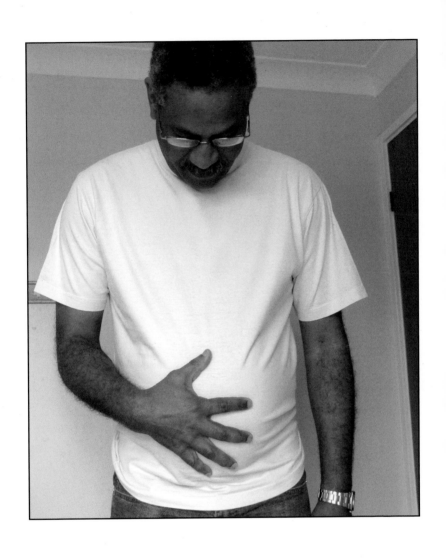

But the pounds come back.
Al weighs more than before!

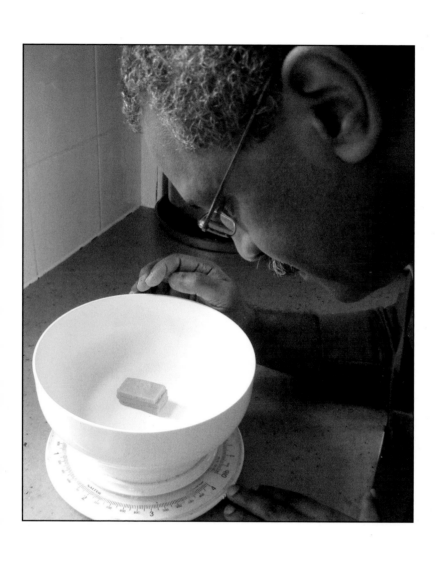

Al tries another diet.

He weighs his food.

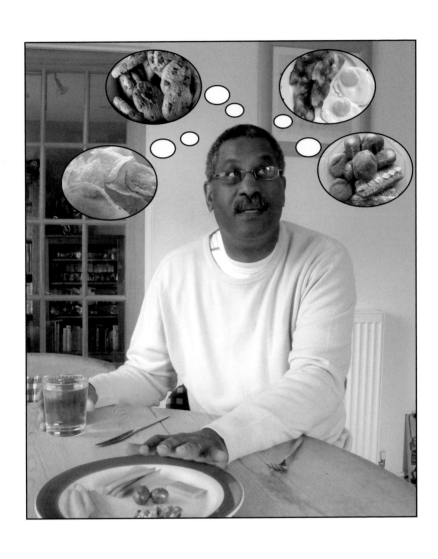

Al eats very little.

He is hungry all the time.

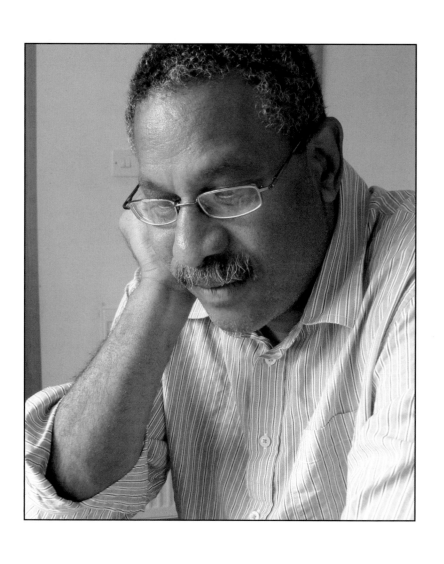

He is tired and cranky all the time.

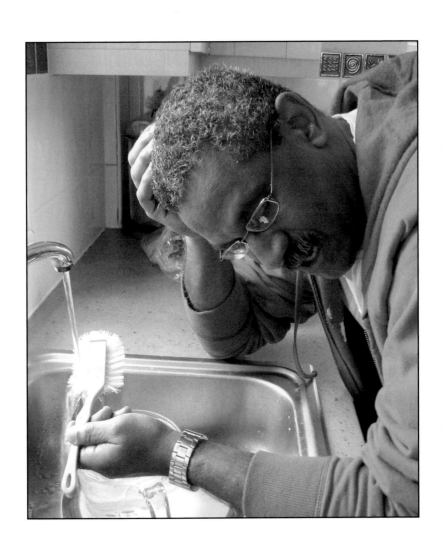

Sometimes Al feels dizzy.

He thinks, "This is crazy!"

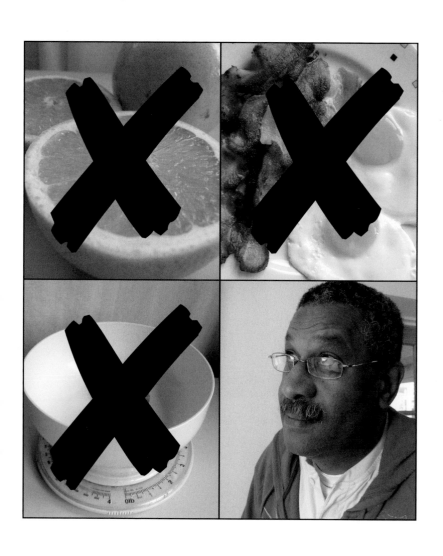

Al learns a lesson.

Fad diets do not work.

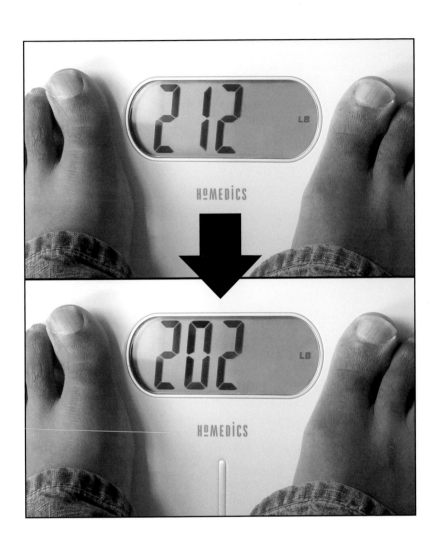

Fad diets promise,
"Lose weight fast!"

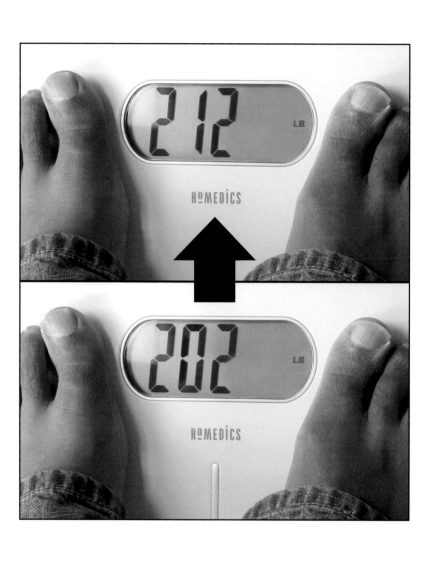

But the weight comes back fast.

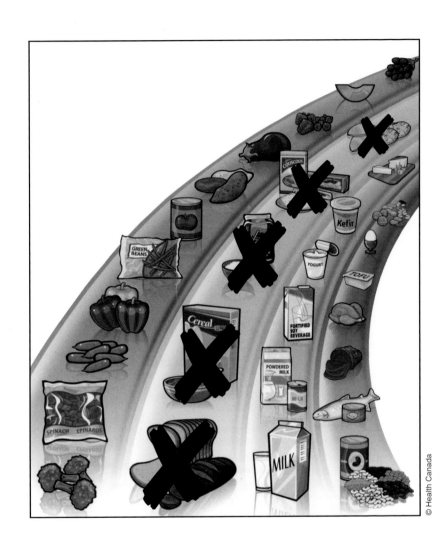

© Health Canada

Fad diets cut out a food group.

This can make you feel tired or sick.

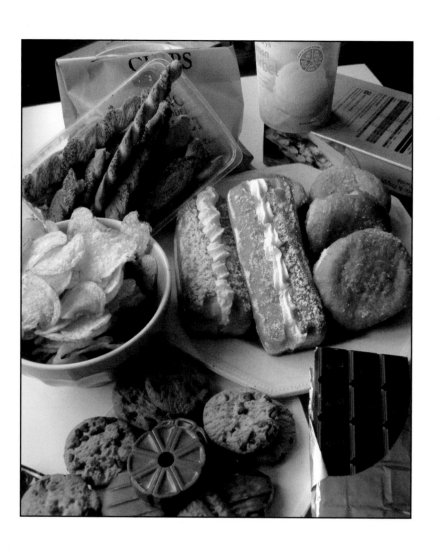

Fad diets make you feel hungry.
So you eat junk food to feel full.

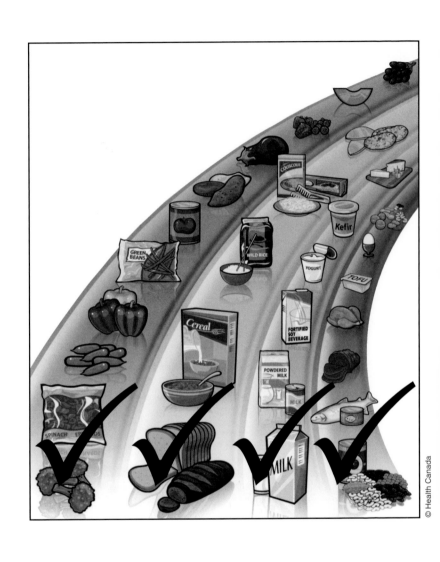

Al starts to eat right.

He eats good food.

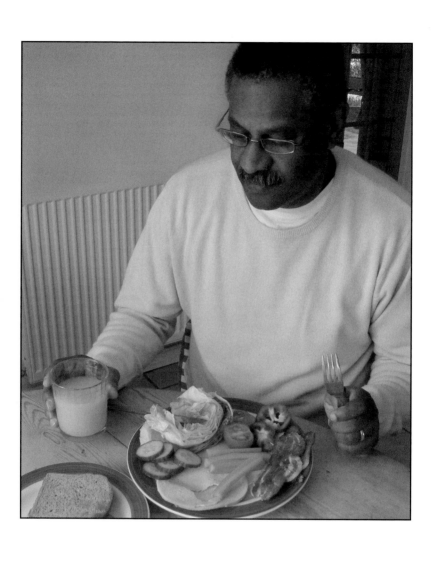

Al eats enough food.

He does not feel hungry all the time.

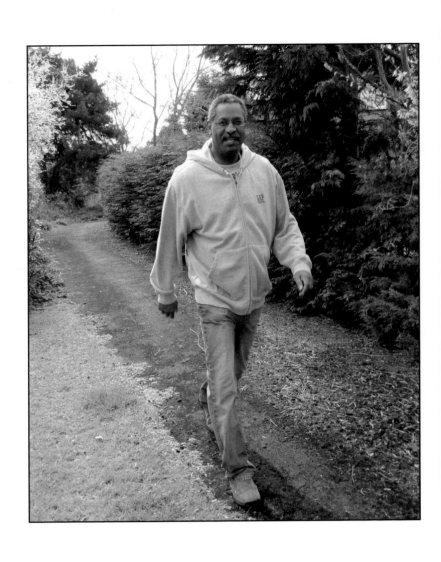

Al starts to exercise more.

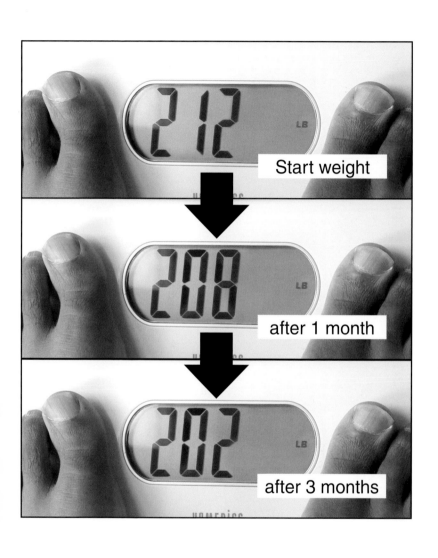

Start weight

after 1 month

after 3 months

Al loses weight safely.

He loses weight little by little.

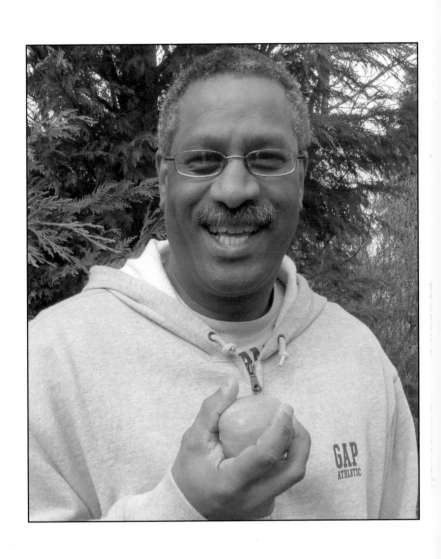

Al feels better.

And he looks better.